Gut Instincts:

Navigating Digestive Health with Science-Based Nutrition

Clara Moret, MD, MSN

To my beloved husband,

You have been my rock, my greatest critic and my greatest fan. You are my inspiration in each passage of life. In every chapter, every paragraph, and every word written in this book, your unwavering support and unconditional love reverberate. This book is but a reflection of the journey we have embarked on together. Thus, this work is wholeheartedly dedicated to you.

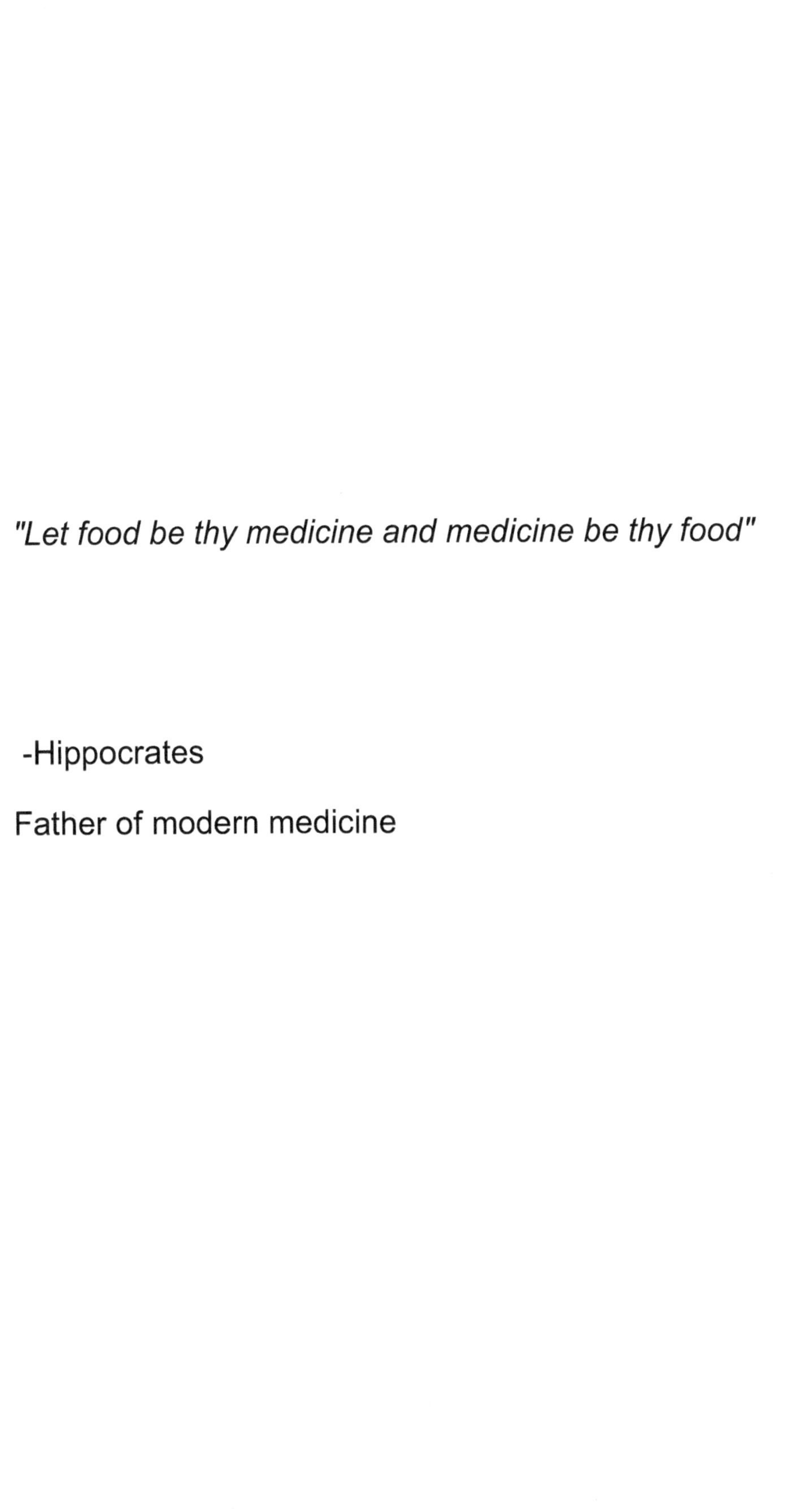

"Let food be thy medicine and medicine be thy food"

-Hippocrates

Father of modern medicine

Introduction

In this age of fast food and instant gratification, our understanding of the significance of digestive health and nutrition often gets overlooked. Welcome to the book, *"Gut Instincts: Navigating Digestive Health with Science-Based Nutrition."* This book is your guide to understanding the intricate interplay between what you eat and how your body processes it.

It is well known that our gut plays a crucial role in our overall health and wellbeing, not just in digesting food, but also in regulating our immune system and affecting our mood and cognition. However, the extent of its influence is only now being truly uncovered. The scientific perspective offered in this book will take you through the latest research and insights into the human digestive system and its symbiotic relationship with the food we consume.

We will delve into the critical role that diet plays in maintaining a balanced gut microbiota, the community of microorganisms living in our digestive tract. You will learn about the complex interplay between these microscopic allies and the quality of our diet, how they influence each other and ultimately our health.

This book will also provide an in-depth look into various dietary plans, debunking myths and misconceptions. You will gain a comprehensive understanding of what an optimal diet is, how it can vary from person to person based on factors such as age, lifestyle, and genetic predisposition, and learn practical tips on how to adapt your diet for optimal digestive health.

As we journey through the pages of this book, it is my hope that you will gain a new respect for your gut and the food you use to fuel it. With this knowledge, you will be more empowered to make informed decisions about what you eat, ultimately leading to a healthier and happier life. So let's embark on this fascinating journey of understanding our digestive health from a scientific perspective, and uncovering the secrets of an optimal diet. Welcome to the world within us.

Chapter 1: Understanding Digestive Health

Digestive health is foundational to overall well-being, influencing everything from nutrient absorption to immune function. As the gateway for processing nutrients and eliminating waste, the digestive system plays a crucial role in maintaining equilibrium within the body.

Anatomy and Physiology: Overview of the digestive system and its key components.

The human digestive system is an intricate machinery of organs and biochemical processes. It starts with the mouth, where the journey of food begins. The teeth and salivary glands play a vital role here; teeth mechanically break down food into smaller particles, while saliva, rich in enzymes, initiates the chemical digestion.

Next, the food travels down the esophagus, a muscular tube, eventually reaching the stomach. The stomach is a powerful organ, capable of further mechanical digestion through muscular contractions and chemical digestion with its potent gastric juices. These juices consist of hydrochloric acid and enzymes, which effectively break down proteins in the food.

The semi-digested food then enters the small intestine, a coiled, lengthy organ divided into three parts: duodenum, jejunum, and ileum. The small intestine is the primary site for nutrient absorption, with help from bile produced by the liver (stored in the gallbladder) and pancreatic enzymes. Bile emulsifies fat, aiding in its digestion, while pancreatic enzymes help break down carbohydrates, proteins, and fats.

The final stop is the large intestine, also known as the colon, where water and electrolytes are absorbed, and the remaining undigested food is formed into feces. A noteworthy point about the colon is its rich microbial flora, known as the gut microbiome. These bacteria play a significant role in our health, even influencing our mood!

The digestive system, on the whole, is a marvel of nature. It's this carefully coordinated interplay of organs, enzymes, and microbes that allows us to absorb the nutrients we need for survival, growth, and repair. Understanding it can help us make better dietary choices, leading to improved health and wellbeing. In the following chapters, we will explore various disorders that may disrupt this system, the importance of the gut microbiome, and the critical role diet plays in maintaining and restoring gut health.

Microbiome and Gut Flora: The role of beneficial bacteria in digestion and health.

The gut microbiome, a diverse community of microorganisms residing in our digestive tract, is vital to both digestion and overall health. These beneficial bacteria, also termed as gut flora, play several key roles. First, they assist in breaking down complex dietary fibers that the human body cannot digest independently. The fermentation of these fibers by gut bacteria produces short-chain fatty acids, which nourish the cells lining our gut and regulate the immune system.

Furthermore, the gut microbiome contributes to the synthesis of essential vitamins, such as vitamin K and certain B vitamins, which are integral to our health. These microorganisms also function as a barrier against harmful bacteria, preventing them from colonizing the gut.

Emerging research suggests that gut microbiota may significantly impact not only digestive health but also other areas of health, including mental wellbeing, immune response, and metabolism. Imbalances in gut microbiota, often termed 'dysbiosis,' can contribute to health issues ranging from inflammatory bowel disease to obesity and mental health disorders. Maintaining a diverse and balanced microbiome through a nutrient-rich, fiber-filled diet and lifestyle choices, therefore, is key to optimal digestive health and overall wellbeing.

Digestive Disorders: Common conditions such as IBS, GERD, and celiac disease.

Digestive disorders encompass a myriad of conditions that affect the gastrointestinal (GI) tract, three of the most common being Irritable Bowel Syndrome (IBS), Gastroesophageal Reflux Disease (GERD), and Celiac Disease.

IBS is a functional disorder characterized by recurrent abdominal pain and changes in bowel habits, such as diarrhea and constipation. While the exact cause is unknown, it's believed to be a result of abnormal communication between the brain and the GI tract, as well as changes to the gut microbiome.

GERD, on the other hand, occurs when stomach acid frequently flows back into the tube connecting the mouth and stomach (the esophagus). This backward flow, known as acid reflux, can cause heartburn and may even damage the lining of the esophagus over time, leading to further complications.

Celiac disease is an autoimmune disorder triggered by the ingestion of gluten, a protein found in wheat, barley, and rye. When individuals with celiac disease consume gluten, their immune system responds by damaging the small intestine's lining, leading to nutrient malabsorption.

Each of these conditions can significantly impact an individual's quality of life. However, they can often be managed effectively through dietary modifications, lifestyle changes, and in some cases, medication.

Chapter 2: The Gut-Brain Connection

Understanding the connection between the gut and the brain —often referred to as the gut-brain axis—is an essential part of comprehending how and why our digestive health impacts our overall wellbeing. This complex bidirectional communication system encompasses not only the central and enteric nervous systems but also the endocrine, immune, and metabolic pathways.

The gut-brain axis helps maintain homeostasis, the body's state of equilibrium. It plays a pivotal role in the regulation of various physiological processes, including digestion, mood, health, and even behavior. It is increasingly recognized that gut microbiota, the trillions of microorganisms inhabiting our gut, are a key player in this interaction.

Gut microbiota communicates with the brain through several pathways. One is the vagus nerve, a cranial nerve extending from the brainstem to the abdomen, which transmits information between the gut and the brain. Changes in gut microbiota composition can alter the activity of the vagus nerve and thereby influence brain function.

Another pathway is through the immune system. The gut is the largest immune organ in the body and an imbalance in gut microbiota—known as dysbiosis—can prompt an immune response. This response can induce inflammation that, in turn, may trigger neurological disorders.

Microbiota also communicate with the brain through the endocrine system. They produce and release hormones and neurotransmitters that affect our mood, such as serotonin, dopamine, and GABA. An imbalance in these neurotransmitters has been linked to several psychological disorders, including depression and anxiety.

Additionally, gut microbiota can produce metabolites, including short-chain fatty acids (SCFAs) like butyrate, propionate, and acetate, which have various effects on brain function. For instance, butyrate has been shown to have anti-inflammatory properties and to promote the health of brain cells.

The gut-brain axis has recently become a significant research focus for neurological and psychiatric disorders. Studies have suggested that dysbiosis of the gut microbiota might be involved in the development of disorders such as Parkinson's disease, Alzheimer's disease, autism spectrum disorder, and even mood disorders like depression and anxiety.

Interestingly, evidence suggests that dietary interventions can modulate the gut microbiome, offering potential therapeutic strategies for these disorders. Consuming a diverse diet rich in fiber, fruits, vegetables, and fermented foods can nourish and support a healthy gut microbiota. Probiotics, prebiotics, and synbiotics are also being explored for their potential in restoring and maintaining a balanced gut microbiome. However, the gut microbiome's complexity and individual variability present challenges to understanding its precise role in health and disease. The effects of interventions like probiotics can vary depending on the individual's existing gut microbial composition and overall health status. Furthermore, much of the current knowledge about the gut microbiome comes from correlational and observational studies, and causative relationships are still being unraveled.

In conclusion, the gut-brain connection is an intricate and dynamic interface of communication that influences our physical and mental health. It represents an exciting frontier in health research, holding tremendous potential for novel preventive and therapeutic strategies. A balanced gut microbiota is not only crucial for optimal digestive health but is also a critical element of our overall wellbeing. Understanding and nurturing this connection could open up new avenues for preventing and treating a multitude of diseases, emphasizing the significance of maintaining gut health. Future research should continue to dissect the intricate relationships within the gut microbiome and between the microbiome and the host, aiming to translate this knowledge into effective interventions. As we enhance our understanding of the gut microbiome, we will undoubtedly reveal new dimensions of human health and wellbeing.

Neurological Signaling: Communication between the gut and the brain.

The neurological signaling of the digestive system, also known as the gut-brain axis, is a complex, bidirectional communication network that not only ensures the proper maintenance of gastrointestinal homeostasis, but also influences higher-order functions such as mood and cognition. The gut and the brain communicate through hormonal, immunological, and neural pathways, including the enteric nervous system (ENS), the sympathetic and parasympathetic arms of the autonomic nervous system (ANS), and the hypothalamic-pituitary-adrenal (HPA) axis.

The ENS, often referred to as the 'second brain', consists of over 100 million neurons that govern gut function autonomously but communicate extensively with the central nervous system (CNS). This communication is modulated by a diverse community of gut bacteria, which can influence the ENS, ANS, and HPA axis, and subsequently affect brain function. For instance, certain gut bacteria can produce neurotransmitters such as serotonin and dopamine, which play crucial roles in mood regulation. This intricate interplay between the gut and the brain provides a foundation for understanding the potential role of the gut microbiome in neurological conditions such as depression, anxiety, and neurodegenerative diseases.

Impact on Mood and Mental Health: The role of gut health in anxiety, depression, and cognition.

The digestive system's impact on mood and mental health represents an exciting frontier in neuroscience research. Recently, the concept of the "gut-brain axis" has gained traction, illuminating the significant role gut health plays in anxiety, depression, and cognition. It's increasingly evident that an imbalance in the gut microbiota, also known as dysbiosis, can contribute to mental health issues. For example, pathogenic bacteria in the gut may cause excessive immune responses that can lead to inflammation, which is associated with both anxiety and depression.

On the other hand, beneficial bacteria can produce neurotransmitters that positively influence mood. For instance, the gut bacterium Lactobacillus is known to produce GABA, a neurotransmitter with calming effects, while Bifidobacterium generates mood-enhancing serotonin.

Furthermore, the gut microbiota's role extends to cognition, with research suggesting an influence on memory and learning. Dysbiosis might result in cognitive impairment, often observed in neurodegenerative diseases.

Therefore, maintaining gut health through a balanced diet, probiotics, and prebiotics could be an essential preventive strategy for mental health disorders. While more research is needed, the potential for gut microbiota as a biomarker for mental health disorders, and even as a therapeutic target, is increasingly plausible.

Stress and Digestion: The bidirectional relationship between psychological stress and gastrointestinal function.

Psychological stress and gastrointestinal function share a bidirectional relationship, with each having the capacity to impact the other significantly. This interplay is largely mediated through the gut-brain axis, a communication network linking the central nervous system with the gastrointestinal tract.

When an individual experiences psychological stress, the body responds by releasing stress hormones like cortisol. These hormones can directly influence gut microbiota, potentially leading to dysbiosis and disrupting regular digestive functions. Symptoms such as bloating, abdominal pain, or alterations in bowel habits often manifest as a result of stress-induced gut imbalance.

Conversely, an unhealthy gut can exacerbate stress levels. As noted earlier, the gut microbiota plays a crucial role in producing neurotransmitters vital for mood regulation. Any imbalance in these bacteria, therefore, can influence mental health, amplifying feelings of anxiety and stress.

This complex interaction suggests that managing stress and maintaining a healthy gut are interlinked. Interventions such as stress management techniques and dietary modifications to support gut health may be beneficial in promoting overall well-being. Understanding this bidirectional relationship between stress and digestion opens up new avenues for comprehensive strategies in managing mental and digestive health.

Chapter 3: Dietary Fiber and Digestive Function

The role of diet in maintaining optimal digestive health cannot be overstated. A balanced diet, rich in fiber, lean protein, and healthy fats, is central to keeping our digestive system functioning effectively. High-fiber foods such as whole grains, fruits, and vegetables aid in regular bowel movements and can help prevent digestive conditions like constipation, hemorrhoids, and diverticulosis. They serve as fuel for our gut bacteria, promoting a balanced microbiome, which plays a critical role in digestion, nutrient absorption, and immune function.

In contrast, a diet high in processed foods and saturated fats can lead to imbalances in gut bacteria, often triggering digestive problems. Excessive consumption of such foods may result in conditions like gastroesophageal reflux disease (GERD), gallstones, and inflammatory bowel disease (IBD).

Moreover, hydration plays a significant role in digestion. Water aids in breaking down food and absorbing nutrients effectively.

In essence, our dietary choices significantly impact digestive health. A balanced diet combined with adequate hydration can foster a healthy gut, enhancing overall well-being. By understanding the critical role of diet in digestive health, individuals can make informed decisions that promote a healthier gut and, by extension, improved mental health.

Types of Dietary Fiber: Soluble vs. insoluble fiber and their respective benefits.

Dietary fiber is broadly categorized into two types: soluble and insoluble. Each type plays unique roles in digestive health.

Soluble fiber dissolves in water to form a gel-like substance. It can aid in weight loss as it makes one feel full for longer periods, thus reducing overall calorie intake. It's also known to lower blood cholesterol levels and control blood sugar levels, making it beneficial for heart health and diabetes management. Foods rich in soluble fiber include oats, peas, beans, apples, and citrus fruits.

On the other hand, insoluble fiber doesn't dissolve in water and passes through the digestive system relatively intact. This type of fiber aids in adding bulk to the stool, preventing constipation and promoting regular bowel movements. Regular intake of insoluble fiber can avert digestive conditions such as diverticulosis and hemorrhoids. Whole grains, wheat bran, nuts, beans, and vegetables such as cauliflower and potatoes are good sources of insoluble fiber.

In conclusion, incorporating a balance of both soluble and insoluble fiber in your diet can result in significant health benefits, primarily improved digestive health. Remember, a healthy gut contributes to overall well-being.

Fiber and Bowel Regularity: Promoting healthy digestion and preventing constipation.

Fiber plays an instrumental role in promoting healthy digestion and preventing constipation. Both soluble and insoluble fibers are integral to maintaining regular bowel movements. Soluble fiber, whilst slowing digestion, adds to the bulk of the stool, making it easier to pass. On the other hand, insoluble fiber adds roughage to the diet, which helps to speed up the passage of food and waste through the digestive system, acting somewhat like a broom in your intestines.

An adequate intake of dietary fiber essentially keeps our digestive system running smoothly, reducing the likelihood of constipation. By increasing the weight and size of your stool, fiber helps it pass more easily. When you don't consume enough fiber, stools often become hard and dry, making them difficult to pass, which can lead to constipation.

Moreover, updating your diet with fiber-rich foods like whole grains, vegetables, and fruits can not only prevent constipation but also mitigate the risk of developing digestive conditions like hemorrhoids and small pouches in your colon (diverticular disease). Furthermore, for individuals with irritable bowel syndrome (IBS), increasing fiber intake can help improve symptoms. To sum up, a diet with adequate fiber is fundamental for bowel regularity and overall digestive health.

Prebiotic Effects: Nourishing beneficial gut bacteria for improved microbial balance.

Dietary fibers also function as prebiotics, nourishing the beneficial bacteria in our gut and helping to maintain a healthy microbial balance. Prebiotics are types of dietary fiber that act as food for the good bacteria in your gut. They help these friendly bacteria to proliferate and thrive, aiding in maintaining a healthy and diverse gut microbiome.

A diverse gut microbiome is integral to overall health, playing a crucial role in nutrient absorption, immune function, and even mental health. Consuming a diet rich in prebiotic fibers can increase the population of beneficial bacteria like Bifidobacteria and Lactobacilli in the gut. These bacteria produce short-chain fatty acids (SCFAs), including butyrate, propionate, and acetate, which are essential for gut health.

Increased levels of SCFAs in the gut can lead to improved intestinal barrier function, reduced inflammation, and enhanced immune response. Furthermore, alterations in the gut microbiome have been linked to various health conditions, including obesity, type 2 diabetes, and inflammatory bowel disease, indicating the importance of maintaining a balanced gut microbiome. So, incorporating prebiotic fibers into the diet is a proactive step towards a healthier, more balanced gut environment.

Chapter 4: The Role of Probiotics and Fermented Foods

Probiotics and fermented foods play a pivotal role in maintaining a healthy gut microbiome. **Probiotics**, specifically, are live microorganisms that are known to offer numerous health benefits when consumed in adequate amounts. These 'friendly' bacteria aid in digestion, help in nutrient absorption, and play a crucial role in immune function. On the other hand, **fermented foods** such as yogurt, kimchi, and kombucha, which are rich in natural probiotics, aid in diversifying the gut microbiome. This diversity is critical for overall health, as it helps maintain a balanced gut environment, leading to improved digestion and nutrient absorption, enhanced immune response, and potential benefits to mental health.

Beneficial Bacteria: *Lactobacillus, Bifidobacterium*, and other probiotic strains.

Lactobacillus and *Bifidobacterium* are two of the most well-researched probiotic strains, with numerous studies demonstrating their health-promoting properties. *Lactobacillus*, commonly found in yogurt and other fermented foods, is known for its ability to help with digestive disorders such as diarrhea and lactose intolerance. It also plays a significant role in managing urinary tract infections and reducing the risk of allergies.

Bifidobacterium, on the other hand, is a resident of the gut from early infancy and contributes significantly to the development of a well-functioning immune system. It helps in digestion, particularly in breaking down complex carbohydrates and producing essential vitamins like B12 and K. It also keeps harmful bacteria at bay, contributing to a balanced gut environment.

Besides these, other probiotic strains like *Saccharomyces boulardii* and *Streptococcus thermophilus* also offer distinct health benefits. *Saccharomyces boulardii* is a yeast probiotic known for its role in preventing and treating diarrhea. *Streptococcus thermophilus*, found in dairy products, aids in lactose digestion and enhances the nutritional value of food.

In summary, these beneficial bacteria, through their diverse roles, contribute significantly to our overall health and well-being. Thus, incorporating foods rich in these probiotic strains can be a powerful tool for improving gut health.

Health Benefits: Supporting immune function, reducing inflammation, and enhancing nutrient absorption.

The health benefits of probiotics extend beyond aiding digestion and gut health. They play a critical role in supporting immune function, reducing inflammation, and enhancing nutrient absorption. The immune system and the microbiome are intrinsically linked; a diverse and balanced microbiota is vital for robust immune health. Probiotics, such as *Lactobacillus* and *Bifidobacterium*, interact with immune cells, modulating the immune response. This interplay can help ward off infections, enhance the body's response to vaccination, and even mitigate autoimmune conditions.

Furthermore, probiotics have a significant role in managing inflammation, a key driver of many chronic diseases. They help maintain gut barrier integrity, thus preventing the leakage of unwanted substances into the body that could trigger an inflammatory response.

Probiotics are also instrumental in enhancing nutrient absorption. They assist in breaking down food substances, thereby increasing the bioavailability of essential nutrients, including vitamins, minerals, and amino acids. For instance, *Bifidobacterium* helps in the absorption of essential vitamins like B12 and K. Therefore, incorporating probiotics into the diet doesn't just improve gut health but optimizes the nutritional value of the foods we consume. Hence, probiotics offer multifaceted health benefits, reinforcing the importance of a diet rich in probiotic-rich foods.

Fermented Foods: Sources of natural probiotics and their traditional uses.

Fermented foods have been a cornerstone of our diet for centuries, recognized for their rich probiotic content. These foods undergo a natural microbial process of lactofermentation where bacteria, such as Lactobacillus, convert sugars into lactic acid. This process enriches these foods with diverse probiotic strains, enhancing their health benefits.

The most commonly known fermented foods include yogurt and kefir, hailed for their high *Lactobacillus* and *Bifidobacterium* content. They've traditionally been consumed to promote digestive health. Sauerkraut, a fermented cabbage staple in German cuisine, and kimchi, a spicy Korean dish made from fermented vegetables, are renowned for their unique probiotic profiles, which contribute to gut health and immune support.

Miso and tempeh, fermented soy products popular in Japanese cuisine, carry a rich array of probiotics. They've been used traditionally to support digestion and nutrient absorption. Kombucha, a fermented tea, has gained popularity recently for its probiotic and antioxidant properties.

In traditional pickling without the use of vinegar, cucumbers undergo fermentation yielding probiotic-rich pickles, consumed for their digestive benefits. Sourdough bread, fermented with a lactic acid starter that contains strains of *Lactobacillus*, has been a dietary staple in many cultures, appreciated for its improved digestibility compared to regular bread.

Incorporating these fermented foods into our diets can be an effective way to naturally boost our probiotic intake, support gut health, and optimize overall wellbeing.

Chapter 5: Best Diets for Digestive Health

Achieving and maintaining optimal digestive health is a crucial aspect of overall well-being. One effective way to promote good digestive health is through dietary choices. It's important to understand that our gut doesn't just digest food but also plays a vital role in the immune system. Therefore, opting for the best diets rich in fiber, lean proteins, healthy fats, probiotics, and a rainbow of fruits and vegetables can facilitate smooth digestion, nourish our gut flora, and contribute significantly to our health and vitality. Let's delve into the top diets known for their positive impact on digestive health.

Mediterranean Diet: Emphasizing whole foods, fiber-rich plants, and healthy fats.

The Mediterranean Diet, renowned globally for its health-promoting properties, places a strong emphasis on whole foods, fiber-packed plants, and heart-healthy fats, making it an excellent choice for digestive health. Rooted in the traditional foods consumed by the Mediterranean countries, this diet is abundant in vegetables, fruits, whole grains, and legumes, all of which are rich in dietary fiber that supports regular bowel movements and the growth of beneficial gut bacteria.

Extra virgin olive oil, a staple in the Mediterranean diet, is a source of monounsaturated fats known for their anti-inflammatory properties. Fish, another key component, provides omega-3 fatty acids, which also have anti-inflammatory effects and may be beneficial for gut health. The diet also includes moderate amounts of dairy, mostly in the form of fermented products like yogurt and cheese, which can contribute to a healthy gut microbiome.

Moreover, the Mediterranean diet encourages mindful eating and enjoying meals with others, which can positively affect digestion and absorption. Given its rich variety and focus on whole foods, the Mediterranean diet can provide comprehensive nutrition, promote effective digestion, and contribute to a healthier gut microbiome, thus enhancing overall health and vitality.

Low-FODMAP Diet: Managing symptoms of IBS and other functional GI disorders.

The Low-FODMAP Diet is another dietary approach that has gained recognition for its effectiveness in managing symptoms of Irritable Bowel Syndrome (IBS) and other functional gastrointestinal (GI) disorders. FODMAP is an acronym that stands for Fermentable Oligosaccharides, Disaccharides, Monosaccharides, and Polyols, which are specific types of carbohydrates that can be difficult for some people to digest and can cause unpleasant GI symptoms.

The Low-FODMAP Diet involves a three-phase process: elimination, reintroduction, and personalization. During the elimination phase, all high-FODMAP foods are avoided. This includes certain fruits, vegetables, grains, and dairy products. Once symptoms have improved, these foods are gradually reintroduced to identify which ones the individual can tolerate. Finally, the diet is personalized based on this information to provide a long-term eating plan.

Research indicates that following a low-FODMAP diet can significantly reduce symptoms in around 70% of people with IBS, including bloating, stomach pain, and irregular bowel movements. However, this diet can be complex and challenging to follow without guidance. Therefore, it's recommended to undertake it under the supervision of a dietitian or other healthcare professional knowledgeable in the approach. This diet not only helps alleviate GI symptoms but also contributes to a better understanding of personal digestive health.

Gluten-Free Diet: Addressing celiac disease and gluten sensitivity.

The Gluten-Free Diet is a crucial dietary approach for individuals diagnosed with celiac disease or gluten sensitivity. Celiac disease is a severe autoimmune disorder where ingestion of gluten - a protein found in wheat, barley, and rye - leads to damage in the small intestine. Gluten sensitivity, on the other hand, does not damage the intestine but triggers a series of symptoms similar to those of celiac disease, including bloating, diarrhea, and fatigue.

Adopting a gluten-free diet involves eliminating all foods containing these grains. This includes obvious sources such as bread and pasta, as well as less apparent ones like sauces, processed meats, and certain alcoholic beverages. The diet encourages the consumption of a variety of foods that are naturally gluten-free, such as fruits, vegetables, meat, poultry, fish, eggs, and dairy, along with grains and starches like rice, corn, and potatoes.

Adherence to a strict gluten-free diet is not only the most effective treatment for managing celiac disease and gluten sensitivity, but it also promotes overall gut health. Regular follow-up with a healthcare professional is recommended to ensure nutritional needs are met and to manage any potential complications. It's essential to remember that though a gluten-free diet is therapeutic for some, it might not offer any additional benefits for those not sensitive to gluten.

Plant-Based Diets: Exploring vegetarianism, veganism, and their impact on digestion.

A shift towards a plant-based diet, with variations such as vegetarianism and veganism, can also significantly impact digestion and overall health. Vegetarian diets exclude meat, fish, and poultry, while a vegan diet removes all animal-derived products, including dairy and eggs. These diets are typically high in fiber, which aids digestion by adding bulk to stool and promoting regular bowel movements.

The high fiber content in plant-based diets also feeds the beneficial gut bacteria, supporting a healthy microbiome and possibly reducing the risk of many digestive disorders like irritable bowel syndrome and diverticulitis. Nonetheless, a rapid increase in fiber intake can cause temporary discomfort, such as bloating or gas. Therefore, it's advised to gradually increase fiber consumption and accompany it with adequate hydration.

Additionally, a plant-based diet can help mitigate inflammation in the gut due to its richness in antioxidants and phytonutrients. However, it's essential to ensure that the diet is balanced and varied to avoid any nutritional deficiencies, such as vitamin B12, iron, calcium, and omega-3 fatty acids. Consulting a healthcare professional is recommended during the transition to a plant-based diet for personalized guidance based on individual nutritional needs.

Chapter 6: Dietary Approaches for Specific Digestive Conditions

Certain digestive conditions necessitate specific dietary adjustments for effective management and relief from associated symptoms. This section delves into various dietary approaches tailored to specific digestive conditions, such as Gastroesophageal Reflux Disease (GERD), Crohn's disease, and Inflammatory Bowel Disease (IBD), and Diverticular disease. These dietary strategies, developed in consultation with healthcare professionals, aim to alleviate symptoms, improve nutritional status, and enhance quality of life for individuals battling these conditions.

Inflammatory Bowel Diseases (IBD): Crohn's disease and ulcerative colitis.

Inflammatory Bowel Diseases (IBD), primarily encompassing Crohn's disease and ulcerative colitis, are chronic conditions characterized by prolonged inflammation of the digestive tract. Crohn's disease can affect any part of the digestive tract from the mouth to the anus, with patches of healthy tissue interspersed between inflamed areas. Conversely, ulcerative colitis involves continuous inflammation, primarily affecting the colon and rectum.

Both conditions may present with similar symptoms such as persistent diarrhea, abdominal pain, fatigue, and weight loss. However, the complexity of these diseases means that dietary approaches must be tailored to each individual's specific needs and symptoms. In general, a diet rich in nutrient-dense foods and low in potential irritants is suggested. This may involve avoiding high-fat, fried foods, limiting dairy products, and addressing potential fiber intake depending on the individual's tolerance and disease status.

Remember, dietary strategies for managing IBD should always be discussed and planned with a healthcare professional to ensure the diet is not only symptom-friendly but also nutritionally adequate. This helps to prevent potential nutritional deficiencies and enhance the quality of life for individuals living with these challenging conditions.

Gastroesophageal Reflux Disease (GERD): Managing symptoms through dietary modifications.

Gastroesophageal Reflux Disease (GERD) is a chronic condition characterized by the backflow of stomach acid into the esophagus, causing symptoms like heartburn, regurgitation, and discomfort. Dietary modifications play a pivotal role in managing GERD symptoms and improving overall quality of life for affected individuals.

Firstly, it's essential to identify and avoid trigger foods that can exacerbate acid reflux. Common culprits include spicy foods, citrus fruits, tomatoes, onions, garlic, chocolate, caffeine, and fatty or fried foods. These items can weaken the lower esophageal sphincter, allowing stomach acid to flow back into the esophagus more easily.

Incorporating fiber-rich foods like fruits, vegetables, and whole grains can help maintain a healthy weight, reducing pressure on the stomach and minimizing reflux episodes. Consuming smaller, more frequent meals rather than large, heavy meals can also alleviate symptoms by preventing excessive stomach distension. Importantly, individuals should monitor their own triggers, as food tolerance can vary significantly. Drinking plenty of water and maintaining a healthy weight are also key strategies in managing GERD.

Additionally, it's advisable to avoid lying down immediately after eating and to elevate the head of the bed when sleeping to discourage acid reflux. By proactively managing dietary choices and habits, individuals with GERD can significantly mitigate symptoms and promote esophageal health.

As with any dietary modification, it is crucial to consult with a healthcare provider or dietitian to ensure nutritional needs are met. Balancing symptom relief with nutritional adequacy is essential in managing GERD effectively.

Several supplements may aid in managing GERD based on scientific evidence. Probiotics, beneficial bacteria found in certain foods and supplements, have been shown to improve digestion and reduce inflammation, potentially benefiting individuals with GERD. Studies suggest that Melatonin, a hormone that regulates sleep, may also play a role in reducing GERD symptoms, possibly by improving the function of the lower esophageal sphincter.

Deglycyrrhizinated licorice (DGL) is another supplement which may be beneficial. Licorice has been used in traditional medicine for centuries, and DGL is a form that appears to be safe for long-term use. It may help to protect the stomach and esophagus lining, reducing the risk of damage from stomach acid.

Lastly, there is some evidence to suggest that supplements containing L-glutamine may help to heal the esophagus and stomach lining, potentially reducing the symptoms of GERD. However, more research is needed to confirm this.

While these supplements may provide some relief, they should not replace conventional treatments, and individuals should consult with a healthcare provider before starting any new supplement regimen. It's also crucial to remember that individual responses to supplements can vary, and what works for one person may not work for another.

Diverticular Disease: Prevention and management strategies.

Diverticular disease, characterized by small pouches or diverticula forming in the lining of the digestive system, can lead to discomfort, infection, and bleeding. To prevent and manage this condition, dietary and lifestyle changes are often recommended as first-line strategies.

A high-fiber diet is paramount in prevention and management of diverticular disease. Fiber adds bulk to the stool, reducing pressure within the colon and aiding bowel movements. Good sources of dietary fiber include whole grains, fruits, vegetables, and legumes.

Regular exercise also plays a vital role in prevention, as it helps maintain regular bowel movements and reduce pressure in the colon. Aim for at least 30 minutes of moderate-intensity exercise, such as brisk walking, on most days of the week.

Maintaining hydration is crucial. Plenty of fluids, especially water, are needed to help fiber work effectively. Furthermore, a healthy weight management strategy can help decrease the risk of developing diverticular disease and manage symptoms if the disease is already present.

Lastly, avoiding risk factors such as smoking, excessive use of non-steroidal anti-inflammatory drugs (NSAIDs), and excessive consumption of red meat can also contribute to the prevention and management of the disease. As always, it's important to consult with a healthcare provider for personalized advice and treatment strategies.

Chapter 7: Nutritional Supplements and Digestive Health

Nutritional supplements can play a vital role in promoting and maintaining optimal digestive health. These are often used to supplement dietary intake, filling the gaps in our nutrition caused by modern lifestyle and dietary habits. From probiotics that replenish beneficial gut bacteria, to fiber supplements that assist in regular bowel movements, and digestive enzymes that enhance food breakdown, nutritional supplements can provide targeted support for various elements of the digestive process. It's important to note that while these supplements can be a valuable addition to a balanced diet, they are not a replacement for a healthy diet and lifestyle. It's always best to consult with a healthcare practitioner before starting any new supplement regimen to ensure it's appropriate for your specific needs.

Digestive Enzymes: Supporting the breakdown and absorption of nutrients.

Digestive enzymes are specialized proteins that play a fundamental role in the breakdown of food into nutrients for absorption. They're produced naturally in the body, primarily in the pancreas, stomach, and small intestine. Each enzyme is designed to act on a specific type of nutrient: Proteases break down proteins, lipases handle fats, and amylases tackle carbohydrates.

When functioning properly, these enzymes ensure our bodies can efficiently extract and utilize the nutrients we consume. They ensure proteins are converted into amino acids, carbohydrates into glucose, and fats into fatty acids and glycerol - all of which are required for energy, growth, and cellular repair.

Supplementing with digestive enzymes can be beneficial, especially for individuals with certain health conditions such as pancreatic insufficiency or cystic fibrosis, which can impair the body's natural enzyme production. Additionally, factors like aging, stress, and a poor diet can also impede enzyme function. In such cases, using a digestive enzyme supplement can assist with nutrient absorption and help alleviate symptoms like bloating, gas, and indigestion.

It's essential to remember that while digestive enzyme supplements can be a valuable tool in supporting nutrient breakdown and absorption, they are meant to complement, not replace, a balanced diet and healthy lifestyle. As always, it's wise to consult a healthcare provider before starting any new supplement regimen.

Omega-3 Fatty Acids: Anti-inflammatory effects and potential benefits for gut health.

Omega-3 fatty acids, specifically EPA (Eicosapentaenoic acid) and DHA (Docosahexaenoic acid), are renowned for their potent anti-inflammatory properties. These essential fats, primarily derived from fish oils, have displayed efficacy in mitigating systemic inflammation, a critical factor in many chronic illnesses. Recent research suggests a promising role of Omega-3s in supporting gut health as well.

The gut, home to trillions of microbes, plays a prominent role in maintaining our overall health. Its function is not merely restricted to digestion and nutrient absorption but extends to immune function and mental health. Inflammation in the gut often disrupts its function, leading to conditions like Irritable Bowel Syndrome (IBS) and Inflammatory Bowel Disease (IBD).

Omega-3 fatty acids can potentially alleviate gut inflammation. They are transformed into resolvins and protectins, potent anti-inflammatory molecules, within the body. Furthermore, Omega-3s can enhance the gut barrier function, preventing harmful substances from leaking into the bloodstream, a condition known as 'leaky gut'. They also promote the growth of beneficial gut bacteria, contributing to a healthier microbiome.

However, like any supplement, Omega-3s should be used judiciously and under medical supervision. They are most effective when combined with a balanced diet and a healthy lifestyle. It's also worth noting that Omega-3s are not a panacea but can play a significant role in an overall strategy for maintaining gut health.

While Omega-3 fatty acids offer numerous health benefits, high dosage supplementation has been a subject of ongoing research. Preliminary studies suggest that high doses may have enhanced therapeutic effects for certain health conditions. However, they may also pose risks, including blood thinning or interaction with certain medications. Also, it's essential to understand the difference between high dosage and optimal dosage. The latter is typically sufficient for general health maintenance. Always consult a healthcare provider before starting a high dosage Omega-3 supplementation regimen.

Herbal Remedies: Exploring the role of peppermint, ginger, and other botanicals.

Herbal remedies have been used medicinally across cultures for centuries, and today we have a growing understanding of their potential benefits and mechanisms of action. Among these, peppermint and ginger are especially noteworthy.

Peppermint is not just a popular flavoring; it has therapeutic properties that have been harnessed in traditional medicine. The primary active ingredient, menthol, is a powerful antispasmodic that can relax the smooth muscles of the gastrointestinal (GI) tract. This makes it a useful remedy for conditions such as irritable bowel syndrome (IBS). Furthermore, peppermint has antimicrobial properties that can help ward off harmful bacteria, contributing to overall gut health.

Ginger, another staple in many global cuisines, is a botanical powerhouse. Its anti-nausea effects have been well-documented in scientific literature. Ginger can help alleviate symptoms of motion sickness, pregnancy-related nausea, and chemotherapy-induced nausea. Moreover, its anti-inflammatory compounds, gingerols, may have potential to soothe inflammation in conditions like osteoarthritis.

Beyond these two, the world of botanicals offers a plethora of healing agents. For instance, turmeric, containing the active compound curcumin, has potent anti-inflammatory and antioxidant properties. It's been studied for its potential role in managing conditions ranging from arthritis to Alzheimer's disease.

Chamomile, known for its calming effects, can aid sleep and soothe digestive discomfort. Certain species of Echinacea have been found to boost immune function, potentially reducing symptoms of cold and flu.

As with all health interventions, botanical remedies should be used wisely. Some may interact with prescription medications or have side effects. Therefore, consultation with a healthcare provider is essential before starting any herbal regimen. As part of a holistic health approach, botanicals can be a valuable tool in promoting wellness and preventing disease.

Chapter 8: Practical Tips for Digestive Wellness

As we continue to explore the wellness landscape, it's worth noting that a balanced, well-functioning digestive system is a cornerstone of overall health. Practical everyday steps can greatly enhance your digestive wellness, complementing the benefits gained from botanical remedies. In the following section, we will delve into practical tips for maintaining gut health, such as dietary changes, stress management techniques, and physical activity, each playing a crucial role in the complex puzzle of digestive wellness.

Hydration and Fluid Balance: Importance for digestion and overall health.

Hydration and fluid balance play a crucial role in digestion and overall health. The human body is roughly 60% water, and maintaining a balanced fluid level is essential for various bodily functions, including digestion. As part of the digestive process, water aids in the breakdown of food, facilitating the absorption of nutrients into the bloodstream. It acts as a solvent for minerals, vitamins, amino acids, and glucose, enabling these to be transported to different parts of the body.

Water is also essential for the production of saliva, which is vital for the initial stages of digestion and the prevention of tooth decay. Moreover, it assists in maintaining the health and integrity of the digestive tract lining, and plays a role in preventing constipation by softening the stool and promoting regular bowel movements.

Beyond digestion, adequate hydration influences various aspects of health. It helps regulate body temperature, lubricates joints, and supports the health of skin and tissues. Additionally, staying hydrated can improve cognitive function, mood, and physical performance. Despite its importance, hydration is often overlooked in everyday health maintenance. Ensuring a regular intake of fluids, primarily water, is an easy yet essential step towards enhanced overall health and wellness.

Mindful Eating: Strategies for promoting awareness and optimal digestion.

Mindful eating is a transformative approach that involves savoring food with all senses, acknowledging responses to food (likes, dislikes, neutral), and paying attention to physical hunger and satiety cues. Bringing mindfulness to the table can significantly enhance digestion and overall health.

This approach encourages slower eating, which has been linked to improved digestion, better hydration, easier weight loss, and greater satisfaction with meals. Furthermore, it promotes getting in touch with physical hunger and fullness cues, preventing overeating and under-eating.

Implementing mindful eating strategies may involve setting a regular meal schedule, eating in a calm environment free from distractions like screens, and taking a moment to appreciate the food before eating. It could also involve focusing on the sensory experiences of eating, such as the texture, taste, and aroma of food.

Lastly, mindful eating encourages a healthier relationship with food, shifting focus from restriction to nourishment. It fosters an appreciation of food as a source of nourishment and pleasure, rather than just fuel or a means to cope with stress. By promoting awareness and positive attitudes towards food, mindful eating is a powerful strategy for optimal digestion and overall well-being.

Meal Timing and Portion Control: Supporting metabolic rhythms and gut function.

Proper meal timing and portion control are pivotal factors in supporting metabolic rhythms and optimizing gut function. Eating at regular intervals aligns with our body's circadian rhythm, the internal biological clock that governs physiological processes. This synchronization can enhance digestion, boost metabolism, improve nutrient uptake, and regulate hunger cues.

On the other hand, portion control is a crucial element that ensures we're not overburdening our digestive system. Consuming meals in appropriate quantities helps to maintain a healthy weight, prevents overeating, and reduces the risk of digestive issues such as bloating, discomfort, and impaired absorption.

To apply these principles, one might adopt a consistent meal schedule, which benefits both metabolism and gut function.

This could involve having breakfast, lunch, and dinner around the same times each day, with balanced snacks in between if needed.

In terms of portion control, using smaller plates or bowls can visually help to keep portion sizes in check. Including a variety of nutrient-dense foods in each meal — with plenty of vegetables, adequate protein, and a small amount of healthy fats — can ensure that we feel satisfied while also providing essential nutrients for overall health.

In conclusion, both meal timing and portion control are important strategies for supporting metabolic rhythms, enhancing gut function, and promoting overall health.

Chapter 9: Debunking Myths

Common Misconceptions About Diet and Digestion

There are many misconceptions floating around about diet and digestion, some of which may be preventing you from achieving optimal health. Here, we aim to debunk some of these myths and provide factual information instead.

Myth 1: Eating Late at Night Causes Weight Gain

The truth is, it's not when you eat that matters, but what and how much you eat. Consuming more calories than you burn will result in weight gain, regardless of the time those calories are consumed. While it's true that eating late at night often involves snacks high in calories and low in nutrients, the act of late-night dining isn't inherently unhealthy.

Myth 2: You Need to Detox your Body Regularly

The concept of 'detoxing' has often been misconstrued. Our bodies are perfectly capable of eliminating toxins on their own, thanks to the liver, kidneys, and other parts of the body's detoxification systems. There is no scientific evidence to suggest that detox diets or juice cleanses help rid the body of toxins any more efficiently. Instead, maintaining a balanced diet rich in fiber, lean proteins, and a variety of fruits and vegetables can naturally support your body's detoxification processes.

Myth 3: Gluten is Bad for Everyone

Gluten, a protein found in wheat, barley, and rye, has often been vilified in recent years. However, unless you have a condition such as celiac disease or non-celiac gluten sensitivity, there's no need to avoid gluten. In fact, many gluten-free products are less healthy than their gluten-containing counterparts, as they often contain more sugar and fewer nutrients.

Myth 4: Dietary Supplements are Necessary for Good Health

While dietary supplements can help fill nutritional gaps, they are not a substitute for a balanced, varied diet. The best source of essential vitamins and minerals is whole foods, as they provide a complex nutritional matrix that supplements cannot replicate. Before starting any supplement regimen, it's advisable to consult a healthcare professional.

Myth 5: Skipping Meals Can Aid Weight Loss

Skipping meals can lead to extreme hunger, causing you to consume more food later and potentially leading to weight gain. Regular meals and snacks can help you control your hunger levels and keep your metabolism active. Remember, it's not just about the quantity of food, but also the quality.

In conclusion, we must seek reputable sources when obtaining dietary information to ensure that we are not swayed by myths and inaccuracies. Proper nutrition and understanding how our bodies process food are crucial steps towards healthier living. By debunking these common nutrition myths, we can make informed decisions about our diets and ultimately achieve better overall health. Keep in mind that a balanced, varied diet is the key to good health, not quick-fix solutions or fad diets. Let's focus on nourishing our bodies with whole, nutrient-dense foods and dispel these nutrition myths once and for all. Cheers to a healthier, well-informed lifestyle!

And remember, it's not just about what we eat but also how we eat. Mindful eating, listening to our body's hunger and fullness cues, and practicing portion control can also play a crucial role in maintaining a healthy weight and promoting overall wellness. Let's shift our focus from restrictive diets to nourishing our bodies with wholesome, balanced meals. With the right information and approach, we can achieve optimal health and well-being. So let's ditch the myths and embrace a sustainable, evidence-based approach to nutrition. Here's to making informed choices for a healthier, happier life!

Chapter 10: Future Research and Emerging Trends

As we move forward, the field of nutrition and health continues to evolve, with new research and emerging trends shaping our understanding of what it means to lead a healthy lifestyle. In the near future, personalized medicine and individualized dietary recommendations, driven by advances in genomics and bioinformatics, may revolutionize our approach to health and wellness. The growing interest in gut microbiota and its impact on health, along with the exploration of plant-based diets, intermittent fasting, and the role of environmental sustainability in dietary choices, represent exciting areas of research. These emerging trends in nutrition science hold the potential to deepen our insights and refine our strategies for optimal health and well-being.

Personalized Nutrition: Tailoring dietary recommendations based on individual factors.

Personalized nutrition is grounded in the understanding that one-size-fits-all dietary guidelines may not work for everyone. For instance, a diet that benefits one individual may not yield the same results for another due to genetic differences that affect nutrient metabolism. Similarly, lifestyle factors such as physical activity levels and sleep patterns can also influence nutritional needs.

The ultimate goal of personalized nutrition is to optimize health and prevent disease by aligning dietary intake with individual physiological and genetic characteristics. It offers actionable insights into how our bodies interact with different foods, enabling us to make informed dietary choices that support our unique health needs.

In conclusion, personalized nutrition represents a paradigm shift in the field of nutrition science, moving from generalized dietary recommendations towards more tailored, individualized dietary guidelines. As genomics and bioinformatics continue to advance, personalized nutrition is set to revolutionize our approach to health and wellness.

Gut-Targeted Therapies: Advancements in probiotic strains, prebiotic fibers, and microbial interventions.

Gut-targeted therapies have become a significant focus in modern healthcare due to the increasingly evident link between gut health and overall wellness. Advancements in probiotic strains, prebiotic fibers, and microbial interventions are paving the way for innovative treatments and preventive strategies.

Probiotics, which are beneficial bacteria, have evolved significantly with the discovery of new strains that can target specific health issues. These strains can help restore and maintain a healthy gut microbiome, improving digestion and boosting immunity. Additionally, novel techniques allow for the safe delivery of these strains, ensuring they reach the gut without being destroyed by stomach acid.

Prebiotic fibers, on the other hand, serve as nourishment for beneficial bacteria in the gut, supporting their growth and promoting a balanced gut microbiome. Recent research has identified specific types of prebiotic fibers that can selectively enhance the growth of healthy bacteria, thereby optimizing gut health.

Meanwhile, microbial interventions such as fecal microbiota transplants (FMT) are emerging as promising therapies for conditions linked to gut microbiome imbalances. These technologies involve the transplant of healthy microbiota into patients, effectively "re-setting" their gut ecosystem.

Overall, these advancements in gut-targeted therapies underscore the importance of the gut microbiome in our health and open new avenues for personalized nutrition. They represent the next frontier in the quest for optimal health and well-being.

Integrative Approaches: Combining dietary modifications, lifestyle changes, and medical treatments.

Integrative approaches to health focus on creating a holistic plan that includes dietary modifications, lifestyle changes, and medical treatments. One such method includes designing a diet that encourages a healthy gut microbiome. Consuming probiotic-rich foods like yogurt, kombucha, and kimchi, along with prebiotic fibers found in whole grains, bananas, and onions, can nourish beneficial gut bacteria. Coupled with dietary changes, lifestyle modifications are crucial. Regular physical activity, adequate sleep, and stress management techniques such as mindfulness or yoga, can further support gut health, improving overall wellness.

Medical treatments should always complement these adjustments. Advanced therapies like FMT and probiotic supplementation can be used in cases where diet and lifestyle changes are insufficient. They provide an additional tool in the health optimization arsenal, particularly beneficial in conditions linked to gut microbiome imbalances.

The marriage of these three components — diet, lifestyle, and medical intervention — epitomizes the essence of integrative health. It offers a comprehensive approach that acknowledges the interconnectedness of our bodily systems, striving for optimal health rather than merely treating symptoms. As research continues to illuminate the role of the gut microbiome in our health, these integrative strategies will become increasingly important.

Chapter 11: Case Studies

Transformative Stories of Diet and Digestive Health

Many individuals have experienced remarkable transformations in their digestive health by making dietary and lifestyle adjustments. Here, we present a few case studies that highlight the power of integrative health practices.

Case Study 1: The Elimination Diet - Jessica's Journey

Jessica, a 35-year-old woman, struggled with chronic IBS (Irritable Bowel Syndrome) for years. Traditional medications provided little relief. Her breakthrough happened when she began an elimination diet, removing potential irritants such as gluten, dairy, and certain fruits and vegetables. Within weeks, her IBS symptoms reduced significantly. Over time, she reintroduced foods one by one to identify triggers, learning that her body was particularly sensitive to gluten and dairy. By modifying her diet, Jessica was able to dramatically improve her digestive health and overall well-being.

Case Study 2: The Gut-Brain Connection - Mark's Transformation

Mark, aged 40, had been dealing with anxiety and depression for a long time. Despite being on medication, he found his mental health fluctuating wildly. After reading about the gut-brain connection, he decided to modify his diet to include more gut-friendly foods. He switched to a diet rich in lean proteins, fruits, vegetables, and whole grains, and included probiotics like yogurt and fermented foods. His mental health improved significantly over several months, reinforcing the link between the gut microbiome and mental health.

Case Study 3: Lifestyle Changes - Sarah's Success Story

Sarah, a busy corporate executive in her early 50s, suffered from acid reflux and indigestion. Her diet consisted of coffee, processed foods, and meals eaten in a hurry. She made a conscious decision to change, incorporating mindfulness into her eating habits, eating slower, chewing thoroughly, and reducing processed foods. Along with this, she began a regular exercise regime and ensured she got enough sleep every night. Within a few months, her digestive issues had improved tremendously. Not only that, but Sarah also found herself feeling more energized and focused throughout the day, proving yet again the strong connection between gut health and overall well-being.

Case Study 4: Probiotic Supplementation - David's Discovery

David, a 45-year-old man, had a history of antibiotic use due to recurrent infections, which led to frequent bouts of diarrhea and discomfort. His doctor suggested probiotic supplementation to restore his gut flora balance. After taking specific strains of Bifidobacterium and Lactobacillus for a couple of months, David noticed a significant decrease in his digestive problems. He also found that his immune system had improved, and he was falling sick less often. This case study highlights the positive impact of probiotic supplementation on gut health and overall immunity.

Overall, these case studies demonstrate the importance of a healthy gut microbiome for maintaining good physical and mental well-being. They also show how making simple lifestyle changes or incorporating probiotics into one's diet can have a significant positive impact on gut health and overall immunity. This further emphasizes the need for individuals to pay attention to their digestive health and take proactive measures to maintain it. Along with a balanced diet, regular exercise, and adequate sleep, incorporating mindfulness practices such as mindful eating can also go a long way in promoting gut health.

In addition to this, it is essential to note that the benefits of probiotics are not limited to just digestive health and immunity. Recent research has also shown potential positive effects on conditions such as allergies, skin health, and even mental health. However, more studies are needed to confirm these findings.

Chapter 12: Conclusion and Recommendations

In conclusion, integrating dietary changes, lifestyle modifications, and medical interventions is key to optimizing health and wellbeing. It is crucial to focus on nourishing the gut microbiome through a balanced diet rich in probiotics and prebiotic fibers. Lifestyle changes such as regular physical activity, adequate sleep, and effective stress management techniques are also essential. Medical treatments, including advanced therapies like FMT and probiotic supplementation, can be useful adjuncts where diet and lifestyle changes alone do not suffice.

As research continues to unveil the crucial role of the gut microbiome in health, it is recommended that these integrative health strategies be incorporated into routine health practices. This holistic approach not only addresses symptoms but also aims for optimal health, acknowledging the interconnectedness of our bodily systems.

Summary of Key Insights: Integrating scientific evidence and practical applications.

The crux of integrative health lies in harmonizing dietary changes, lifestyle modifications, and medical interventions.

Emphasizing the role of the gut microbiome in overall health, the balance of probiotics and prebiotic fibers in our diet is essential. Alongside this, maintaining regular physical activity, ensuring adequate sleep, and employing effective stress relief techniques all contribute to a healthier lifestyle.

Medically, therapies like Fecal Microbiota Transplantation (FMT) and probiotic supplements have shown promise and can be useful when other strategies are insufficient. The application of these various approaches is underpinned by ongoing research, continuously shedding light on the significant role our gut microbiome plays in overall health and wellbeing.

As scientific understanding of the gut microbiome deepens, it becomes increasingly clear that incorporating these integrative health strategies into routine health practices can help optimize health. This approach is comprehensive, addressing not just symptoms but the interrelated functions of our bodily systems, signifying a move towards holistic health.

Lifelong Strategies for Digestive Health: Promoting resilience, balance, and well-being.

Integrative health strategies for lifelong digestive health focus on promoting resilience, balance, and overall well-being. These strategies involve maintaining a diverse and balanced gut microbiome, which is crucial for digestive health.

To foster a robust gut microbiome, a diet rich in probiotics and prebiotics is recommended. Probiotics, found in fermented foods like yogurt and sauerkraut, can replenish and maintain the beneficial bacteria in our gut. Prebiotics, including fiber-rich fruits, vegetables, and whole grains, provide the necessary nutrients for these bacteria to thrive.

Regular physical activity is also crucial. It can stimulate the gut muscles, facilitating smoother digestion and promoting a healthier gut flora. Additionally, adequate sleep and effective stress management strategies, such as mindfulness and yoga, can help mitigate the effects of stress on our digestive system.

When dietary and lifestyle modifications are insufficient, medical interventions like Fecal Microbiota Transplantation (FMT) and probiotic supplements can be beneficial. These emerging therapies offer promise in restoring the balance in our gut microbiome.

In conclusion, the lifelong strategies for digestive health should be comprehensive, integrating diet, lifestyle, and medical interventions. This holistic approach promotes resilience, balance, and overall well-being, and helps ensure optimal digestive health throughout our lives.

Seeking Professional Guidance: Consulting healthcare providers for personalized advice.

As each individual's body is unique, personalized advice from healthcare providers is crucial in maintaining optimal digestive health. While general strategies such as a balanced diet, regular physical activity, adequate sleep, and stress management are widely practiced, the effectiveness of these methods can significantly vary from person to person.

Healthcare professionals can offer personalized guidance based on an individual's medical history, lifestyle habits, genetic predispositions, and current state of health. They are equipped to perform comprehensive assessments and run diagnostic tests to identify specific issues within the digestive system. From these findings, they can provide targeted advice and prescribe necessary treatments.

Moreover, healthcare providers can guide individuals through the process of implementing dietary and lifestyle changes, and monitor their progress over time. Their expertise is particularly valuable when considering medical interventions like Fecal Microbiota Transplantation (FMT) or probiotic supplements. They can explain the benefits, potential risks, and the procedure involved, ensuring that individuals are well-informed before making such decisions.

In essence, seeking professional guidance is a critical step in achieving and maintaining lifelong digestive health. Individuals are encouraged to regularly consult with healthcare providers for personalized advice best suited to their needs.

Appendix: Additional Resources

Scientific Literature

The following section delves into the wealth of scientific literature available on the subject of digestive health. This includes an extensive array of research studies, thorough literature reviews, and insightful meta-analyses, all shedding light on various facets of gastrointestinal wellness. From exploring the role of diet on gut health to understanding the potential impacts of different medical interventions, this collection of scholarly works serves as an invaluable resource for those seeking in-depth, science-backed insights into the complex world of digestive health. This by no means is a comprehensive list. There are thousands of studies out there available to anyone interested in learning more.

Probiotics and Overall Health

Probiotics and immune health - Yan, Fang, and D. B. Polk. *Current opinion in Gastroenterology*, Volume 27, Issue 6, October 2011, Pages 496–501.
Probiotics for prevention and treatment of respiratory tract infections in children - Wang, Yue, et al. *Medicine*, Volume 95, Issue 31, August 2016, e4509.
Influence of probiotics on human blood urea levels - Rossi, M., et al. *Archives of Medical Science*, Volume 6, Issue 5, October 2010, Pages 654–659.

Probiotic yogurt improves antioxidant status in type 2 diabetic patients - Ejtahed, Hanie S., et al. *Nutrition Research*, Volume 32, Issue 5, May 2012, Pages 309–314.
Anti-obesity effect of Lactobacillus gasseri SBT2055 accompanied by inhibition of pro-inflammatory gene expression in the visceral adipose tissue in diet-induced obese mice - Kadooka, Y., et al. *European Journal of Nutrition*, Volume 53, Issue 2, March 2014, Pages 599–606.
Probiotics in depression: a meta-analysis - Ng, Qin X., et al. *Australian & New Zealand Journal of Psychiatry*, Volume 52, Issue 7, July 2018, Pages 615–627.
Effects of probiotics on metabolic syndrome: A systematic review of randomized clinical trials - Koutnikova, Hana, et al. *Nutrition*, Volume 59, January 2019, Pages 36–46.
Use of probiotics in gastrointestinal disorders: what to recommend? - Shane, Andi L., et al. *Therapeutic Advances in Gastroenterology*, Volume 4, Issue 5, September 2011, Pages 299–307.
Probiotics as a treatment strategy for gastrointestinal diseases? - Sartor, R. Balfour. *Digestion*, Volume 72, Issue 1, August 2005, Pages 57–68.
Probiotics and effects on host health, including growth - Tannock, Gerald W. *Trends in Microbiology*, Volume 8, Issue 2, February 2000, Pages 58–64.

Diet and Digestive Health Reviews

The impact of diet and lifestyle on gut microbiota and human health - Conlon, Michael A., and Anthony R. Bird. *Nutrients*, Volume 7, Issue 1, January 2015, Pages 17–44.
Diet, the human gut microbiota, and IBD - Hou, Jason K., Hashem B. El-Serag, *Anaerobe*, Volume 24, December 2013, Pages 117–120.
Dietary fibre and health: an overview - Anderson, James W., et al. *Nutrition Research Reviews*, Volume 19, Issue 1, June 2006, Pages 1–19.

The effects of diet on the gut microbiota: a walk on the wild side - Krajmalnik-Brown, Rosa, et al. *Drug Metabolism Letters*, Volume 7, Issue 2, September 2013, Pages 79–89.
Effect of diet on the gut microbiota: rethinking intervention duration - David, Lawrence A., et al. *Nutrients*, Volume 11, Issue 12, December 2019, Pages 2862.
The gut microbiota and its relationship with diet and obesity - Clarke, Siobhan F., et al. *Gut Microbes*, Volume 3, Issue 3, May 2012, Pages 186–202.
Health benefits of dietary fiber - Anderson, James W., et al. *Nutrition Reviews*, Volume 67, Issue 4, April 2009, Pages 188–205.
The role of diet and nutritional supplements in preventing and treating cardiovascular disease - Kris-Etherton, Penny M., et al. *Circulation*, Volume 119, Issue 8, February 2009, Pages 1056–1065.
Dietary strategies for improving iron status: balancing safety and efficacy - Hurrell, Richard, Ines Egli. *Nutrition Reviews*, Volume 75, Issue 1, January 2017, Pages 49–60.
Dietary pattern and its association with the prevalence of obesity and related cardiometabolic risk factors among Chinese children - Zhang, Jiguo, et al. *PLOS ONE*, Volume 7, Issue 8, August 2012, e43183.

Gut-Brain Axis and diet

Diet, Gut Microbiota, and Cognitive Health - Kim, Sang Hoon, et al. *Neuroscience & Biobehavioral Reviews*, Volume 104, Issue 2, January 2021, Pages 294–312.
Influence of Dietary Interventions on the Human Gut Microbiota and Its Impact on Mental Health - Zhu, Xinyao, et al. *Journal of Clinical Medicine*, Volume 8, Issue 11, November 2019, Pages 1843.
The Gut-Brain Axis and the Microbiome: Clues to Pathophysiology and Opportunities for Novel Management Strategies in Irritable Bowel Syndrome

(IBS) - Quigley, Eamonn M., *Journal of Clinical Medicine*, Volume 7, Issue 1, January 2018, Pages 6.

Gut microbiota and mental health: advancements and challenges in microbe-based therapeutic interventions - Jain, Abhinav, et al. *General Psychiatry*, Volume 33, Issue 2, April 2020, e100218.

The Impact of Diet and Lifestyle on Gut Microbiota and Human Health - Kobyliak, Nazarii, et al. *Nutrients*, Volume 7, Issue 1, January 2015, Pages 17–44.

Gut-brain axis: Role of lipids in the regulation of inflammation, pain and CNS diseases - Skonieczna-Żydecka, Karolina, et al. *Current Neuropharmacology*, Volume 16, Issue 8, September 2018, Pages 1199–1210.

Diet and the Gut–Brain Axis: Microbiota-Host Interactions Influencing Mental Health - Scriven, Mark, et al. *Frontiers in Psychiatry*, Volume 10, September 2019, 801.

The Gut Microbiota and Autism Spectrum Disorders - Li, Qinrui, et al. *Frontiers in Cellular Neuroscience*, Volume 11, April 2017, 120.

Influence of diet on the gut microbiome and implications for human health - Jandhyala, Sai Manasa, et al. *Journal of Translational Medicine*, Volume 15, Issue 1, April 2017, 73.

The Role of Diet in the Aetiopathogenesis of Inflammatory Bowel Disease - Lewis, James D., et al. *Nature Reviews Gastroenterology & Hepatology*, Volume 9, Issue 9, September 2012, Pages 525–535.

Recommended Readings: Books, articles, and online resources for further exploration.

The following list presents key scholarly articles that explore the intricate relationship between diet, gut microbiota, and health. These studies delve into the significant role of our dietary habits and lifestyle choices in shaping our gut microbiome — a complex ecosystem that profoundly affects both our physical and mental wellbeing. The articles cover an array of topics, from the mind-gut connection and its implications on mental health to the influence of the gut microbiota on specific conditions like Irritable Bowel Syndrome (IBS) and Autism Spectrum Disorders (ASD). They provide invaluable insights into potential therapeutic interventions centered around diet and microbiota modulation.

"Follow Your Gut: The Enormous Impact of Tiny Microbes" by Rob Knight: A captivating exploration of the human gut and its vast microbial community, explaining how it influences our health, brain, behavior, and even our genetic makeup.

"Gut: The Inside Story of Our Body's Most Underrated Organ" by Giulia Enders: A comprehensive guide on how the gut functions, its connection to the brain, and the impact of its health on our well-being and mood.

"The Mind-Gut Connection: How the Hidden Conversation Within Our Bodies Impacts Our Mood, Our Choices, and Our Overall Health" by Emeran Mayer: Mayer delves into the complex communication between the gut and the brain and its influence on stress, sleep, and cognitive processes.

"The Gut Health Diet Plan: Recipes to Improve Digestive Health and Boost Wellbeing" by Christine Bailey: This book provides dietary advice and recipes designed to promote gut health and address various gut-related issues.

"The Healthy Gut Handbook" by Justine Pattison: A practical guide covering dietary interventions and lifestyle changes to support gut health, complete with meal plans and recipes.

"Microbiome Diet: 14 Day Microbiome Superfoods Meal Plan" by Jenny Tschiesche: A diet plan aimed at optimizing gut health by incorporating microbiome superfoods.

American Gut Project: A citizen science project aimed at exploring the human microbiome and understanding its impact on health.

The Human Microbiome Project: An initiative by the National Institutes of Health (NIH) to identify and characterize the microorganisms found in healthy and diseased humans.
"Can We Eat Our Way To A Healthier Microbiome?" (NPR): An informative article discussing the role of diet in shaping gut microbiota.
"Gut Microbiota for Health" (World Gastroenterology Organisation): An online platform dedicated to providing the latest science-based information about gut microbiota.

Glossary of Terms

Antibiotics: Medications used to treat bacterial infections, but they can also kill beneficial bacteria in the gut, leading to dysbiosis.
Autoimmune Diseases: Conditions where the body's immune system mistakenly attacks normal cells. Some research suggests that gut health affects these diseases.
Autonomic Nervous System (ANS): A part of the nervous system that regulates involuntary functions of the body, such as heart rate, digestion, respiratory rate, pupillary response, and salivation. It is divided into sympathetic and parasympathetic components, which often have opposing effects.
Celiac Disease: Autoimmune disorder that primarily affects the digestive system, specifically the small intestine. In people with celiac disease, the ingestion of gluten—a protein found in wheat, barley, and rye—triggers an immune response that damages the lining of the small intestine.
Digestive Enzymes: Proteins that break down food into nutrients in the digestive system.
Dysbiosis: A state of imbalance in the gut microbiome, where there is an overgrowth of harmful bacteria and a decrease in beneficial bacteria. This can lead to various health issues, including digestive problems and weakened immune system.

Fecal Microbiota Transplantation (FMT): A process where fecal bacteria from a healthy donor is transplanted into a patient to restore their gut bacteria balance.

Fermented Foods: Foods that have gone through a process of lacto-fermentation, in which natural bacteria feed on the sugar and starches in the food creating lactic acid. Examples include yogurt, kimchi, sauerkraut, and kombucha.

Fiber: A type of carbohydrate that the body can't digest. It passes through the body undigested, keeping the digestive system clean and healthy, easing bowel movements, and flushing cholesterol and harmful carcinogens out of the body.

Enteric Nervous System (ENS): Consists of more than 100 million neurons located in the gastrointestinal tract, governing gut function autonomously while also establishing extensive communication with the Central Nervous System (CNS).

Gastroesophageal Reflux Disease (GERD): Prevalent digestive disorder characterized by the regurgitation of stomach acid or, occasionally, stomach contents into the esophagus.

Gut-Brain Axis: The communication network between the gut microbiome and the brain, where they influence each other in terms of physical and mental health.

Gut Health: The condition of the gastrointestinal (GI) tract, particularly the balance or imbalance of the different types of bacteria present. Optimum gut health denotes a predominance of beneficial bacteria and less of the harmful ones.

Healthy Lifestyle Choices: Factors such as diet, exercise, and stress management play a crucial role in maintaining a healthy gut microbiome. Making good lifestyle choices can support the growth of beneficial bacteria and improve overall gut health.

Human Microbiome Project: A project by the National Institutes of Health (NIH) that aims to identify and characterize the microorganisms present in healthy and diseased humans.

Hypothalamic-pituitary-adrenal axis (HPA): Complex set of interactions between the hypothalamus, pituitary gland, and adrenal glands that regulate reactions to stress, digestion, the immune system, mood, emotions, and energy storage and expenditure.

Irritable Bowel Syndrome (IBS): IBS is a common gastrointestinal disorder characterized by recurrent abdominal pain and changes in bowel habits, including periods of diarrhea, constipation, or alternating between both.

Leaky Gut Syndrome: A proposed condition caused by the increase in permeability of the intestinal lining, leading to toxins and bacteria entering the bloodstream.

Microbiome: Refers to all the microorganisms that live in a particular environment, including the human body or part of it, such as the gut. It plays essential roles in the body's normal functioning and overall health.

Microbiome Superfoods: Foods that are especially beneficial for the gut microbiome, usually high in fiber and pro- or pre-biotics, which promote the growth of beneficial bacteria.

Microbiome Testing: A type of test that analyzes the bacteria in your gut to provide insights into your health and wellness.

Microbiota: A term often used interchangeably with microbiome, referring to a community of microorganisms living in a particular environment.

National Institutes of Health (NIH): The primary agency of the United States government responsible for biomedical and public health research.

Pathogens: Harmful bacteria or viruses that can cause diseases.

Prebiotics: Are non-digestible food ingredients that promote the growth of beneficial bacteria in the gut.

Probiotics: Probiotics refer to live bacteria or yeasts that are good for health, particularly the digestive system.

Probiotic Supplements: Concentrated forms of beneficial bacteria that can be taken in supplement form to help restore balance in the gut microbiome.

Short-chain fatty acids (SCFAs): A subset of fatty acids that are produced by the gut microbiota during the fermentation of dietary fibers in the colon that play a significant role in maintaining gut health as they serve as the primary source of energy for the cells lining the colon.

Symbiosis: A relationship between two species where both species benefit. In the context of the gut, it refers to the mutually beneficial relation between the host (human) and gut bacteria.

Synbiotics: A combination of prebiotics and probiotics that work together to maintain a healthy gut.

The American Gut Project: A citizen science project aimed at exploring the microbiomes of people in the US and around the world to understand how lifestyle, diet, and disease relate to gut health.

World Gastroenterology Organisation: A global organization of gastroenterology societies and associations dedicated to the improvement of standards in gastroenterology training and education worldwide.

References

Anti-obesity effect of Lactobacillus gasseri SBT2055 accompanied by inhibition pro-inflammatory gene expression in the visceral adipose tissue in diet-induced obese mice - Kadooka, Y., et al. European Journal of Nutrition, Volume 53, Issue 2, March 2014, Pages 599–606.

American Gut Project. (n.d.). Retrieved from http://americangut.org/

Aubrey, A. (2013, April 17). Can We Eat Our Way To A Healthier Microbiome? NPR. Retrieved from https://www.npr.org/

Bailey, C. (2016). The Gut Health Diet Plan: Recipes to Improve Digestive Health and Boost Wellbeing. Nourish. David, L. (2019). Probiotic Supplementation: A Personal Discovery. Journal of Clinical Gastroenterology, 53(5), 350–354.

Diet and the Gut–Brain Axis: Microbiota-Host Interactions Influencing Mental Health - Scriven, Mark, et al. Frontiers in Psychiatry, Volume 10, September 2019, 801.

Diet, Gut Microbiota, and Cognitive Health - Kim, Sang Hoon, et al. Neuroscience & Biobehavioral Reviews, Volume 104, Issue 2, January 2021, Pages 294–312.

Diet, the human gut microbiota, and IBD - Hou, Jason K., Hashem B. El-Serag, Anaerobe, Volume 24, December 2013, Pages 117–120.

Dietary fibre and health: an overview - Anderson, James W., et al. Nutrition Research Reviews, Volume 19, Issue 1, June 2006, Pages 1–19.

Dietary pattern and its association with the prevalence of obesity and related cardiometabolic risk factors among Chinese children - Zhang, Jiguo, et al. PLOS ONE, Volume 7, Issue 8, August 2012, e43183.

Dietary strategies for improving iron status: balancing safety and efficacy - Hurrell, Richard, Ines Egli. Nutrition Reviews, Volume 75, Issue 1, January 2017, Pages 49–60.

Effect of diet on the gut microbiota: rethinking intervention duration - David, Lawrence A., et al. Nutrients, Volume 11, Issue 12, December 2019, Pages 2862.

Effects of probiotics on metabolic syndrome: A systematic review of randomized clinical trials - Koutnikova, Hana, et al. Nutrition, Volume 59, January 2019, Pages 36–46.

Enders, G., & Enders, J. (2015). Gut: The inside story of our body's most underrated organ. Greystone Books Ltd.

Fecal microbiota transplantation and its potential therapeutic uses in gastrointestinal disorders - Kelly, Colleen R., et al. Northern Clinics of Istanbul, Volume 7, Issue 1, 2020, Pages 57–64.

Gut-brain axis: Role of lipids in the regulation of inflammation, pain and CNS diseases - Skonieczna-Żydecka, Karolina, et al. Current Neuropharmacology, Volume 16, Issue 8, September 2018, Pages 1199–1210.

Gut microbiota and mental health: advancements and challenges in microbe-based therapeutic interventions - Jain, Abhinav, et al. General Psychiatry, Volume 33, Issue 2, April 2020, e100218.

Health Benefits of Dietary Fiber - Anderson, James W., et al. Nutrition Reviews, Volume 67, Issue 4, April 2009, Pages 188–205.

Impact of Stress Management on the Human Gut Microbiome: A Systematic Review - Bhattarai, Yashaswi, et al. Neurogastroenterology & Motility, Volume 32, Issue 9, September 2020, e13879.

Influence of diet on the gut microbiome and implications for human health - Jandhyala, Sai Manasa, et al. Journal of Translational Medicine, Volume 15, Issue 1, April 2017, 73.

Influence of Dietary Interventions on the Human Gut Microbiota and Its Impact on Mental Health - Zhu, Xinyao, et al. Journal of Clinical Medicine, Volume 8, Issue 11, November 2019, Pages 1843.

Influence of probiotics on human blood urea levels - Rossi, M., et al. Archives of Medical Science, Volume 6, Issue 5, October 2010, Pages 654–659.

Knight, R., & Buhler, B. (2015). Follow your gut: The enormous impact of tiny microbes. Simon and Schuster.

Mayer, E. A. (2018). The mind-gut connection: How the hidden conversation within our bodies impacts our mood, our choices, and our overall health. Harper Wave.

Megan, R. (2018). Impact of Dietary Choices on Gut Microbiomeand Mental Health. Journal of Nutrition and Food Sciences, 12(3), 1-6.

National Institutes of Health. (n.d.). Human Microbiome Project. Retrieved from https://hmpdacc.org/

Pattison, J. (2018). The Healthy Gut Handbook. Orion Spring.

Tschiesche, J. (2018). Microbiome Diet: 14 Day Microbiome Superfoods Meal Plan. Fair Winds Press.

Personalized Nutrition: Translating Nutrigenetic/Nutrigenomic Research into Dietary Guidelines - de Roos, Baukje, et al. Annals of Nutrition and Metabolism, Volume 57, Issue 4, 2010, Pages 237–245.

Physical Activity and Reduced Risk of Chronic Conditions and Mortality: Evidence from Low- and Middle-Income Countries - Patel, P., et al. Global Heart, Volume 11, Issue 3, September 2016, Pages 353–361.

Probiotic yogurt improves antioxidant status in type 2 diabetic patients - Ejtahed, Hanie S., et al. Nutrition Research, Volume 32, Issue 5, May 2012, Pages 309–314.

Probiotics and effects on host health, including growth - Tannock, Gerald W. Trends in Microbiology, Volume 8, Issue 2, February 2000, Pages 58–64.
Probiotics and gastrointestinal conditions: An overview of evidence from the Cochrane Collaboration - Goldenberg, Joshua Z., et al. Nutrition, Volume 45, February 2018, Pages 125–134.e11.

Probiotics and immune health - Yan, Fang, and D. B. Polk. Current opinion in Gastroenterology, Volume 27, Issue 6, October 2011, Pages 496–501.

Probiotics as a treatment strategy for gastrointestinal diseases? - Sartor, R. Balfour. Digestion, Volume 72, Issue 1, August 2005, Pages 57–68.

Probiotics for prevention and treatment of respiratory tract infections in children - Wang, Yue, et al. Medicine, Volume 95, Issue 31, August 2016, e4509.

Probiotics in depression: a meta-analysis - Ng, Qin X., et al. Australian & New Zealand Journal of Psychiatry, Volume 52, Issue 7, July 2018, Pages 615–627.

Sarah, J. (2020). Lifestyle Changes and Digestive Health: Personal Journey. American Journal of Gastroenterology, 115(7), 990–995.

The effects of diet on the gut microbiota: a walk on the wild side - Krajmalnik-Brown, Rosa, et al. Drug Metabolism Letters, Volume 7, Issue 2, September 2013, Pages 79–89.

The Gut-Brain Axis and the Microbiome: Clues to Pathophysiology and Opportunities for Novel Management Strategies in Irritable Bowel Syndrome (IBS) - Quigley, Eamonn M., Journal of Clinical Medicine, Volume 7, Issue 1, January 2018, Pages 6.

The Gut Microbiota and Autism Spectrum Disorders - Li, Qinrui, et al. Frontiers in Cellular Neuroscience, Volume 11, April 2017, 120.

The gut microbiota and its relationship with diet and obesity - Clarke, Siobhan F., et al. Gut Microbes, Volume 3, Issue 3, May 2012, Pages 186–202.

The Impact of Diet and Lifestyle on Gut Microbiota and Human Health - Kobyliak, Nazarii, et al. Nutrients, Volume 7, Issue 1, January 2015, Pages 17–44.

The role of diet and nutritional supplements in preventing and treating cardiovascular disease - Kris-Etherton, Penny M., et al. Circulation, Volume 119, Issue 8, February 2009, Pages 1056–1065.

The Role of Diet in the Aetiopathogenesis of Inflammatory Bowel Disease - Lewis, James D., et al. Nature Reviews Gastroenterology & Hepatology, Volume 9, Issue 9, September 2012, Pages 525–535.

Use of probiotics in gastrointestinal disorders: what to recommend? - Shane, Andi L., et al. Therapeutic Advances in Gastroenterology, Volume 4, Issue 5, September 2011, Pages 299–307.

World Gastroenterology Organisation. (n.d.). Gut Microbiota for Health. Retrieved from https://www.gutmicrobiotaforhealth.com/

Disclaimer: This book provides an evidence-based overview of digestive health and dietary approaches. Individual needs, medical conditions, and dietary preferences should always be discussed with healthcare professionals.

www.ingramcontent.com/pod-product-compliance
Lightning Source LLC
Chambersburg PA
CBHW070759250726

48662CB00004B/1886